Hydroger Health Benefits and Uses

By

Barbara Moore

ISBN-13: 978-1490532165

Table of Contents

Hydrogen Peroxide Health Benefits and Uses

By Barbara Moore

© Copyright 2013 Barbara Moore

First Published, 2013

Printed in the United States of America

Introduction

Hydrogen peroxide or better known as H2O2 is a very common compound that is used to clean and disinfect wounds. It is coupled with betadine solution which cleans wounds and reduces the risk of infection. But what most of us don't know is that the lowly hydrogen peroxide may also be used in other ways and this is due to the efficient properties of this compound.

Hydrogen peroxide appears clear and slightly viscous compared to water in room temperature. This compound is available in opaque plastic bottles and is sold in most drug stores or chemists. Hydrogen peroxide sold in local stores is available as a solution which is partly water. Consumers may be able to purchase hydrogen peroxide in water solutions at 3 to 6% concentrations however there are also commercial grade hydrogen peroxides that are stronger. There are 70 to 98% concentrations which are usually used for industrial purposes and usually require careful packaging and expert handling since these are extremely hazardous. These higher concentrations of hydrogen peroxides are usually used in various industries for cleaning and bleaching; it is also applied to cleaning wastewater in small communities and cities. Some are used for preparing chemicals and for starting chemical reactions. Hydrogen peroxide has so many uses making it one of the most commonly used compounds.

Chapter 1. What is Hydrogen Peroxide Made of

As mentioned, the main reason for the varied uses of hydrogen peroxide is its composition. It is one of the simplest classes of peroxides and its manufacture is usually done through the reaction of oxygen with air as well as organic compounds. Higher compositions of hydrogen peroxide contain stabilizers like phosphates and salts to reduce decomposition while still on storage; hydrogen peroxide will easily decompose into water and oxygen when heat is applied. This compound will also develop into crystalline solids which is why it is used as an oxidizing agent. The most common oxidizing agents from hydrogen peroxide are laundry detergents and bleaches.

Pure hydrogen peroxide is colorless and clear in room temperature; it freezes at temperatures of -0.43 degrees Centigrade and its boiling point is at 150.2 degrees Centigrade. It is soluble in ether and in alcohol. It is viscous and denser than water. Pure peroxide has a pH of 6.2 classifying it as a weak acid; since it is usually diluted in water, its pH levels could be as low as 4.5 at 60% concentrations.

Chapter 2. Brief History of Hydrogen Peroxide

The discovery of hydrogen peroxide is credited to Louis Jacques Thenard in 1818. The chemist created the compound by reacting peroxide (barium peroxide) and an acid (nitric acid). Thenard further used hydrochloric acid with sulphuric acid and this technique was used to create hydrogen peroxide up to the mid-20th century. But before the 21st century, newer and more refined ways of creating hydrogen peroxide was used. Newer techniques also improved productivity and provided better yield of the compound which is extensively used in so many industries all around the world.

The most updated way to manufacture hydrogen peroxide is through the distribution of isomers 2-amyl anthraquinone, a process developed by Solvay, a Belgian chemical company. This chemical process yields pure hydrogen peroxide in 100% concentration.

Chapter 3. Possible Uses of Hydrogen Peroxide

In discussing the use of hydrogen peroxide, it is important to remember that this compound is available in different strengths or concentrations which mean stronger concentrations are commonly used in industrial applications and chemical reactions while weaker concentrations are used in medical facilities and at home.

Cleaning wastewater

The most common problem in wastewater treatment facilities is the terrible smell. When wastewater is processed, hydrogen sulphide is released into the air and this gas is a poisonous and corrosive gas. Hydrogen sulfide or H2S is very strong it can damage wastewater treatment equipment and even solid structures used to contain wastewater sludge. Large concentrations of hydrogen peroxide are added to wastewater to reduce the formation of hydrogen sulfide and leads to the following effects:

1. Wastewater can be treated longer and more efficiently before it can be released at sea or in

specific sewage dumping sites. When wastewater is treated thoroughly, there will be less effect on living things found on sewage dumping areas like remote seas.

2. There will be less damage to the environment when wastewater is treated with hydrogen peroxide since hydrogen sulfide production is minimized. Hydrogen sulfide is strong and corrosive; imagine the environmental damage this gas can do when released in large quantities. Sewage dumping sites will continue to operate and keep the municipality or city clean when efficient wastewater treatment is done.

3. When hydrogen peroxide is used over wastewater, costly equipment used to contain and treat sewage water will be preserved. Treatment plants will operate more efficiently and breakdowns due to faulty equipment will likely be reduced.

Hydrogen peroxide is further used in high strength wastewater treatment because of its efficient oxidizing abilities. It can significantly improve wastewater refinery systems because it is safe and is also very simple to use. Hydrogen peroxide has one of the strongest oxidizing abilities and this property makes it an ideal treatment chemical in various pollutants in water and wastewater.

Hydrogen peroxide can destroy any type of pollutant in wastewater without the need of any additives to facilitate the reaction plus it can be used in any pH levels or wastewater temperatures. When pollutants become harder to oxidize with hydrogen peroxide, iron is often added to create a catalyzed oxidation to destroy pollutants faster and more efficiently.

Industrial bleaching

Tons of hydrogen peroxide is used in the manufacture of paper. When trees are cut to make paper, the pulp or wood is not yet ready to be used. It has to undergo different stages of treatment and one of these is a thorough bleaching process. Wood pulp is naturally grainy and discolored; bleaching whitens it making it look as white as what we know paper to be.

The most common bleaching agent used in this process is alkaline hydrogen peroxide. This type of peroxide is used in bleaching mechanical as well as recycled pulp wherein ink is removed to make fibers of recycled paper brighter.

Chapter 4. Domestic Uses of Hydrogen Peroxide

This chapter will describe and help you to understand various domestic uses of hydrogen peroxide.

Bleaching Human Hair

Hydrogen peroxide is a cheap way to bleach human hair and hence the term "peroxide blonde." The most common dilution used is between 3 to 8% concentrations and is often mixed with ammonium hydroxide. Although there are many hair coloring products available in the market and professional hair coloring treatments, there are a few people who decide to use hydrogen peroxide as an inexpensive way to color hair.

Hydrogen peroxide is easy to use to color hair at home; if you are looking for a straightforward way to bleach your hair without spending too much then follow these simple instructions:

1. Prepare 3% hydrogen peroxide, an empty spray bottle, hair clips, cotton balls and a bath towel for your hair.

2. Wash your hair first and then apply your usual conditioner. Washing your hair will remove all the grime and reduce oil that could interfere with peroxide on your hair.

3. Air dry your hair, do not blow dry or use curling irons.

4. Test the amount of peroxide you will use on your hair by applying a small amount with a cotton ball on some strands of hair.

5. Divide your hair into sections so you can apply peroxide easier. Use hair clips to place hair back and then decide which style you would like on your hair.

You may choose simple highlights on your hair which is done by apply a small amount of hydrogen peroxide in a cotton ball and applying it on hair that you want to color. Start from the root to the tips. After you are finished with one section, you may proceed with the other sections.

If you want the tips to look brighter than the roots then start applying the cotton ball soaked with hydrogen peroxide from the tips towards the roots of the hair strands. But if you want to lighten all your hair then you can spray hydrogen peroxide all over your hair. Use a comb to apply peroxide on all sections of your hair evenly.

6. The golden rule of using hydrogen peroxide on hair is that the longer you let it stay on hair the brighter your hair becomes. And so you need to wait for at least 30 minutes

before rinsing but if you have darker hair then you should allow it to remain on your hair longer.

7. Rinse your hair thoroughly with cold water afterwards; use your usual shampoo and apply hair conditioner afterwards. Make sure you thoroughly rinse peroxide from your hair since having this on your hair for a long time may burn your scalp and damage your hair.

In using hydrogen peroxide to whiten hair, you will be able to achieve your bleached-blonde look after several applications of peroxide. It is natural to notice only minor changes in color on the initial day and you need to repeat this every day or every other day until you have achieved your desired color.

Coloring your hair with hydrogen peroxide is inexpensive indeed but there are some precautions you need to remember. Any chemical or hair treatment that is meant to change the color of your hair could be very hazardous to hair and scalp so be very careful in using these. Experiment on a small section of your hair before using all over your head. And before you start applying on your hair, make sure you set your time and rinse your hair on the expected time to reduce damage.

Hair will become prone to damage every time you use peroxide or other hair coloring treatments so avoid applying heat or using pressure on your hair and scalp. Refrain from using blow dryers, curling irons and flat irons as well as using clips and rubber bands that will only damage hair.

Removing Stains

Since hydrogen peroxide has strong oxidizing abilities, it can remove fresh blood stains on clothes as well as blood stains on other items. This compound is so effective it is also popularly used as a whitening agent in bones of animals and humans that will be placed on display. To use peroxide to remove fresh stains on clothing, just follow these simple tips:

1. Spread the article of clothing with the fresh stain. Rinse the stain with warm water.

2. Allow the warm water to soften the stain for a few minutes then rinse.

3. Place your article of clothing on a small bowl or vat and then apply a generous amount of hydrogen peroxide on the stain. Allow this to sit for about 20 to 30 minutes.

4. After the specified time, use a soft brush to remove the stain. Gently brush the stain away but do not strain the fabric.

5. Use warm water to rinse the fabric. Repeat the procedure if there are still remaining stains.

Hydrogen peroxide is used in removing stains since it does not discolor colored clothes. It is also safe to use so you may use it as a stain remover as much as you want or for as long as the stain remains. Be sure to use 3% hydrogen peroxide concentration and protect your hands as you treat your clothes. For best results, wash treated clothes with cold soapy water afterwards to thoroughly remove the fresh stains or fresh blood stains.

Cleaning Products For Home Use

If you are looking for an alternative and inexpensive home cleaning product that is also very effective then why not use hydrogen peroxide? You may use 3% hydrogen peroxide together with baking soda or vinegar as an alternative cleaning product. Since vinegar has strong oxidizing power, it can efficiently remove stains and dirt from the following surfaces at home:

1. Tile and grout stains – your kitchen and bathroom tiles are very prone to trap dirt and stain because of the use of inefficient cleaning products. Hydrogen peroxide will cut grease and grime and will effectively lift dirt even from the smallest crevices in between tiles to keep these clean. Hydrogen peroxide will never damage delicate tiles even natural stone tiles and will also help maintain the gloss of porcelain tiles.

2. Stainless steel sinks – kitchens and bathrooms which have stainless steel sinks will benefit so much from the oxidizing and cleaning power of hydrogen peroxide especially when combined with baking soda. This mixture is the perfect combination of a homemade cleaning solution that will effectively lift dirt, remove grease and dirt that may settle over the sink and sides and will never damage the sleek and stylish look of stainless steel.

3. Cleaning toilet bowls – just like cleaning tiles and grout, hydrogen peroxide may also be used to clean toilet bowls. Simply spray hydrogen peroxide over your toilet bowl, allow this to settle for 20 to 30 minutes and then flush. You may never need to use elbow grease and other cleaning products to clean anymore.

4. Cleaning tile and natural stone floors – yes hydrogen peroxide is preferred by more and more homeowners in cleaning ceramic and porcelain tile floors as well as natural stone floors. For daily maintenance of these floors a much-lower concentration of hydrogen peroxide should do the trick but for heavily-stained floors you may use 12% solution or a higher concentration. Be sure to be very careful and talk to your floor materials supplier if you can use hydrogen peroxide for your floors or not. This inexpensive and readily available cleaning solution may be done daily since you don't have to worry about damaging your floors.

5. For cleaning burned pots and pans – now you don't need to throw your burned pots and pans away, you may use hydrogen peroxide to remove these burned surfaces easily. Simply mix baking soda and hydrogen peroxide to form a paste, allow this to settle for about 30 minutes. The burned stains will come out when you scrub the pot with dish soap and a sponge.

6. Cleaning and preparing your cutting boards – your cutting boards are just one of the dirtiest surfaces in your kitchen since you usually have time to clean these thoroughly. Before cutting food, especially raw food on your cutting board, spray this with hydrogen peroxide. You will find that the peroxide will bubble indicating that there is bacteria or microbes on the area; allow this to bubble for a few minutes before you scrub the area clean. Rinse your cutting board before cutting food.

7. Cleaning appliance surfaces – you don't notice it but your kitchen is a haven for germs that may cause sickness; the most common areas where microbes settle is on appliance surfaces like your dishwasher, refrigerator, your microwave oven and on any surface on the kitchen counter top. Simply place hydrogen peroxide in spray bottle and then spray on the area you want to clean; let it settle on the area for a few minutes and then wipe it clean. Follow up with a soapy sponge and warm water. You may use this technique every day or when you have extensively used your kitchen appliance for cooking or preparing your food.

8. In washing dishes – when washing dishes that have been stocked for a long time in the cupboard, you may use hydrogen peroxide or with baking soda. Spray a small amount of hydrogen peroxide and allow this to settle on your dishes before rinsing and then washing with dish soap and a sponge. You may also use hydrogen peroxide and baking soda paste on your dishes.

9. Cleaning play areas and toys – since hydrogen peroxide is safe to use, it can be safely used as a surface cleaner over areas where your kids play. Playrooms and nurseries may look unsuspecting but it is one of the best places where microbes and allergens that cause asthma proliferate. Place hydrogen peroxide in a spray bottle and spray this in areas where your kids stay. Allow the peroxide to set on the area before wiping it clean. For very dirty surfaces or when your child has recently been ill, wash the area with water and soap and then allow the area to dry. Spray with hydrogen peroxide and allow this to dry. You may also spray this over stuffer toys, over cribs, cabinets and on walls.

Hydrogen peroxide may be extensively used all over so many areas of your home especially on high traffic areas and in places where dirt and grime accumulate. However, you must remember to take extra precaution in using this in your daily cleaning.

Keep a window open or an exhaust fan open to remove odor that is usually present after using hydrogen peroxide. Using this technique may be very effective but could sting and irritate your hands. Use gloves to work with hydrogen peroxide and remember to wash your hands completely after using this treatment.

Growing Plants

Hydrogen peroxide will help take care of your plants at home. Fungus is the most common parasites that invade plants and these may often destroy plants completely unless controlled. You may use hydrogen peroxide while you water your plants; place this in a spray bottle and spray like you would water on your plants. Spray this over the leaves and the roots of plants. The best concentration is about ½ cup of hydrogen peroxide in a gallon of water.

Horticulturists have studied the use of hydrogen peroxide on plants to improve plant growth. Along with hydroponics, hydrogen dioxide decomposition can release oxygen to enhance root development. This technique may also be used to prevent root clot which is caused by lack of oxygen delivered to the roots, the most distal part of the plants. Plants that were exposed to hydrogen peroxide treatment were seen to grow healthier and stronger roots as well as exposure to hydroponics.

Chapter 5. Therapeutic Use of Hydrogen Peroxide

Hydrogen peroxide has been recognized as a safe oxidizing agent and due to its efficient cleaning and disinfecting properties it has been known to also be used as an antimicrobial compound. In places where sanitation is very important like hospitals, clinics, surgical suites, doctor's offices and other medical treatment facilities, a concentration of 35% hydrogen peroxide is used; this is enough to prevent the spread of microbes and other infectious agents. When hydrogen peroxide comes in contact with a surface, it emits hydrogen peroxide vapor which is a sporicidal sterilant on its own. Here are other therapeutic uses of hydrogen peroxide:

1. Hydrogen peroxide as toothpaste. Hydrogen peroxide is a suitable toothpaste when it is mixed with baking soda and salt, and it may even help to improve the shine or may whiten teeth.

2. Combined with benzoyl peroxide, hydrogen peroxide can be used to treat acne. Acne is the combination of dirt, oil and bacteria creating terrible zits that can lead to

infection and scarring when not treated completely. Hydrogen peroxide will clean and disinfect acne and will help improve wound healing as well.

3. In cleaning wounds, hydrogen peroxide is a cleaning agent that can effectively clean wounds however there are studies that although this compound may be an effective wound cleanser, it may lengthen wound healing time since cells that are repaired are damaged when exposed to hydrogen peroxide. Scarring may also be prevented when peroxide is used therefore it is often omitted when new cells are beginning to form in a wound.

4. Alternative remedies have promoted the use of hydrogen peroxide for the treatment of so many illnesses. There are reports that drinking low concentrations of hydrogen peroxide will help treat cancer however these were all countered by the American Cancer Society saying that cancer treatment should be left to professionals and that there is no evidence that hydrogen peroxide treatment will work on cancer.

Aside from cancer treatment, advocates of hydrogen peroxide treatment have beliefs that this compound may be effective in the treatment of asthma, spinal disease, multiple sclerosis, high blood pressure and leukemia to name a few. However, before considering hydrogen peroxide treatment talk to your doctor beforehand. Your doctor will advise the ideal treatment for your condition after a thorough medical examination and series of diagnostic procedures.

Other uses of hydrogen peroxide

Hydrogen peroxide may also be used as a propellant in rockets and engines. It is also a propellant in thrusters found in satellites. There are some cases that hydrogen peroxide may also be used for making bombs which is why the sale of large quantities and higher concentrations of the compound is strictly regulated.

Special Considerations in The Use of Hydrogen Peroxide

In using hydrogen peroxide, special considerations have to be considered. The safety of the user and the patient for one is one of the most important concerns. Here are some safety concerns in the use of this compound:

1. Hydrogen peroxide is available in very weak concentrations or in very strong and caustic concentrations. Make sure that you are using the correct strength of peroxide that is suitable for your application.

2. In using higher concentrations of hydrogen peroxide, there is a potential risk of suffering from burns. Therefore you should use gloves and protective goggles when handling. If you work in an industry that uses high concentrations of hydrogen peroxide, you should never inhale fumes or directly handle the chemical.

3. Never ingest hydrogen peroxide even if in low concentrations since these may cause burns as well as vomiting and may even lead to death. Do not immediately take oral peroxide as an alternative treatment; taking this orally may only lead to terrible complications.

4. When used as a disinfectant or in cleaning superficial wounds, there is stinging, irritation of the surrounding tissues and redness that will remain on the site for several minutes. Usually wounds may take longer to heal since hydrogen peroxide basically destroys new tissue growth. If your wounds worsen or these side effects persist, discontinue use and contact your doctor. Do not use hydrogen peroxide to clean your wounds unless directed by your doctor.

5. Allergic reactions to hydrogen peroxide is rare but those who do suffer from this condition have symptoms that call for immediate medical action like severe itching on the application site, swelling, development of rash, difficulty in breathing and weakness. Use of peroxide must be discontinued and the person must be taken to an emergency facility as soon as possible.

Chapter 6. Where Do You Purchase Hydrogen Peroxide?

Weak concentrations of hydrogen peroxide may be readily purchased in pharmacies or in drug stores anywhere. Higher concentrations used in medical facilities are usually purchased directly from dealers or manufacturers and a special permit and background checks may be done depending on where you live. Toxic concentrations used for cleaning wastewater and in bleaching are also purchased directly from suppliers and special permits are usually procured to be able to purchase large amounts of hydrogen peroxide.

Conclusion

Learning about many impressive benefits of hydrogen peroxide and some of its disadvantages will allow you to appreciate how a lowly wound cleanser that we knew before has so many uses. It could be useful at home as well as in any industry since it has properties that can clean, disinfect and oxidize which are needed in so many kids of industries and applications.

There are many more uses of hydrogen peroxide however anyone who would like to use it must take extra precaution regarding safety of use and handling. It is also important to be particular about the strength of hydrogen peroxide you are using beforehand to minimize dangerous side effects that are linked to its use. And finally, in using peroxide as an alternative treatment, care should always be exercised. You must talk to your doctor and only follow the recommendations of a professional before taking any medications or treatment; hydrogen peroxide is caustic and will only lead to burns and other dangerous adverse effects when ingested.

Thank You Page

I want to personally thank you for reading my book. I hope you found information in this book useful and I would be very grateful if you could leave your honest review about this book. I certainly want to thank you in advance for doing this.

Printed in Great Britain
by Amazon.co.uk, Ltd.,
Marston Gate.